To
AMERICA
as a
NURSE

To AMERICA *as a* NURSE

SUSAN KAMAU

Copyright © 2014 by Susan Kamau.

Library of Congress Control Number: 2014912921
ISBN: Hardcover   978-1-4990-5316-6
             Softcover   978-1-4990-5315-9
             eBook   978-1-4990-5314-2

All rights reserved. No part of this book may be reproduced or transmitted in any form or by any means, electronic or mechanical, including photocopying, recording, or by any information storage and retrieval system, without permission in writing from the copyright owner.

Any people depicted in stock imagery provided by Thinkstock are models, and such images are being used for illustrative purposes only.
Certain stock imagery © Thinkstock.

This book was printed in the United States of America.

Rev. date: 09/30/2014

To order additional copies of this book, contact:
Xlibris LLC
1-888-795-4274
www.Xlibris.com
Orders@Xlibris.com
642381

TABLE OF CONTENTS

Preface 7

Introduction 9

Chapter 1: NANCY: Relocation and the Transition 13

Chapter 2: URIAH: At the Acme 23

Chapter 3: RICHARD: Making Informed Decisions 30

Chapter 4: SALLY: Accreditation of Schools 35

Chapter 5: ERIC: Gender Based Careers – stereotype
           or reality 40

Conclusion 49

Preface

Every foreign trained nurse has a story to tell about their transitional journey into American nursing, information they wish they would have known prior to flying out, people they wish they would have listened to or not listened to, survival tactics and much more. The highlight of their story is the determination, resilience, discipline that catapulted them to reach their goal.

This book is an informative compilation of stories inspired by experiences of foreign trained nurses during their transitional journey into American nursing. Although the stories in this book have been inspired by true experiences of the nurses, the characters depicted therein are fictional.

The characters in these stories show the challenges and obstacles faced by the transitioning nurses, how they survived the transitional journey and finally became successful nurses in America. Some highlights of the book include: challenges faced by the foreign trained nurse like licensure, finances, choice of friends, source of information, getting accredited institutions of higher learning, importance of giving back to the community, mentoring the young nurses and the challenges male nurses encounter in a female dominated career.

I would like to register my heartfelt gratitude to my family and friends for their enthusiastic encouragement, useful critique, and belief in me throughout the process of writing this book. It was indeed a great journey and your input made it even better. Photography credits to Nyamuwaks and cover page design credits to DLWV creative.

Introduction

"If I could give you information of my life it would be to show how a woman of very ordinary ability has been led by God in strange and unaccustomed paths to do in His service what He has done in her. And if I could tell you all, you would see how God has done all, and I nothing. I have worked hard, very hard and I have never refused God anything."

Florence Nightingale

Growing up, the question "what would you like to be when you grow up?", was dreaded by many. Especially if one did not have a clue of what career path one wanted to take or the career choice was not prestigious or professional enough. Indeed, this was the question one never wanted to answer and tried to avoid at all costs. Family reunions and get togethers were the opportune times relatives and family friends seemed most interested with the grades in school and career ambitions. Unfortunately, these relatives never seemed to forget the fact that one kept changing careers year after year.

One's career path is influenced by the people who cross their life either through the media, in real life or their environment. Some people know their careers right away, while others discover their career after high school, or after going through a life changing moment, or when they see a great need or opportunity in the local and international community or after meeting with a career counselor, or after attending career fair, yet, to others it is a journey that keeps going for a while and we still have others who change their careers three or four times in their life.

Many people, male and female, young and old, fight to ensure they succeed in their careers. There are several motivators to succeed in one's career. These may include but not limited to; passion for the career, success of others in the same career, need for mentors and coaches in their line of practice, monetary gain, job security, job flexibility or by inheritance.

Today's careers have expanded in knowledge, training and technology. Nursing is one of the professions that has seen great changes over the centuries. It has evolved from a home duty, to a vocational skill to a practical skill till today, it is considered one of the most lucrative professions. Nursing has evolved from a skill that was passed down from generation to generation to a fully accredited profession, from following other people's decisions and orders to making their own decisions and orders. The nurses have taken pride in caring for the sick in their homes, in the community, dispensaries, nursing homes, clinics, hospitals, war zones, and refugee camps, with no discrimination of color, gender, race, tribe, or social status. Nursing has also faced many challenges over the years to include shortage, stigmatization, harsh working conditions, fast paced changes in technology, migration of nurses to different countries, brain drain mostly in third world countries amongst others. The Nurse has influenced the level of efficiency of the healthcare system globally. Healthcare is severely affected in places with shortage of nurses.

Factors like missionary work, wars, natural disasters, education, better working conditions, better career opportunities among others have led nurses to migrate from one country to another, from one continent to another. In order to maintain nursing competency every country has a nursing council that gives guidelines on how to practice in that particular country. However, even though a foreign trained nurse has passed the board exam and adheres to the stipulations of nursing practices she/he will still face many challenges while practicing.

Culture shock, strange and mixed traditions, religions, lifestyles, foods, disease and health conditions, climate and strange tongues are but a few of the things that welcomes the foreign trained nurse to a new country or continent. Being prepared and having true facts and ideas of what to expect, eases the anxiety and frustrations that come with migrating from one place to another. Subsequently, the foreign trained nurse is better equipped to face the challenges of being in a foreign land.

This book will take the reader through a simulation journey of the tears, jeers and cheers of a foreign trained nurse relocating to the United States of America and other first world countries through the stories of the characters depicted. It will provide the foreign trained nurse different ways of transitioning into the new nursing system, highlight various challenges and ideas on how to overcome them.

CHAPTER 1
NANCY: Relocation and the Transition

Once you allow yourself to identify with the people in a story, then you might begin to see yourself in that story even if on the surface it's far removed from your situation.

Chinua Achebe

Nursing has a peaceful way of intriguing both adults and children. The noble and professional way nurses present themselves wins the heart of the patients and their families. It is indeed a pleasure to have a nurse by ones bedside. Being the majority in the healthcare system, nurses are in most cases the pace setters of the healthcare system. The good news is that nurses are taught same concepts globally and these concepts can be transferred from one facility to another, one city to the other, one country to the other, one continent to the other.

However, a rift is created due to the adopted and adapted cultures, policies and procedure of the land where one is practicing nursing. An immigrant will have to cross this rift in order to smoothly transition to the next environment. Many people have discovered this rift and there are both fraud as well as faithful people who claim to help foreign trained nurses to transition into the new land.

It is therefore important for the transitioning nurse to be informed about the process. This information will help the nurse save on money, time, energy and emotions. It is also important for the foreign trained nurse to know the culture, equipment, be willing to face obstacles and have enough patience to overcome the frustrations that come with this change.

Nancy

It all started from the doctor's office. Whenever Nancy walked into the doctor's office, she saw the picture of a nurse with a finger on her lips and under the picture was the word SILENCE. This was the quietest place Nancy ever came to, except for the occasional 'maaami!!! Daaady!!! Waahii!! Woowi!!' of babies and children from the injections they were receiving. There would be a group of ladies wearing white dresses, white caps, what looked like very comfortable shoes and a stethoscope hanging round their necks. Nancy never knew who they were so she called them the 'Angels who keep germs away from children'. The most fascinating thing was their smile. Their smile had a way of making the injections seem less painful. Nancy felt good when her 'Angels' would wipe away her tears. This, she believed, made her heal faster.

During one of the school holidays, she went to visit her grandparents. While playing outside, one of her cousins fell and bruised his knee and started crying of pain. Nancy asked her grandfather to take her cousin to the place with the 'Angels'. Her grandfather looked at her grandmother with a worried look and asked Nancy "Who are these Angels?" Nancy, with a wide smile, replied. "The Angels who put on white dresses and white caps and stethoscopes around their neck. They keep the germs and pain away from little children". Her grandmother took her aside and told her, "my child, they have one name, they are called Nurses. Your Auntie Lillian is one of them." Nancy told her grandmother, as sure as the day lights, "when I grow up, I want to be a Nurse. I will be the best, and all the children will love me, and I will keep all germs and pain away from the children, I will wipe their tears and give them a smile." With that, her grandmother blessed her ambition.

As she advanced to higher classes in school, she got a chance to join the Girl Guide club in primary school; where they were taught several things including first aid. She was so good at it that she was always called upon to take care of the injured. She believed it was her smile that healed her classmates. So she always wore it. Nancy was able to proceed to high school and after successful completion, she was admitted to the University and after four years of hard work, and participating in community based health events, she graduated with a Bachelor of Science in Nursing and was very excited for she could not wait to be the 'Angel' she always wanted to be.

After passing her Nursing Council Boards and completing the one year internship at the local hospital, she proceeded to apply for jobs in hospitals and clinics near and far. Eventually, she got a job, her family and friends joined her in praising God and celebrating the victory and toasting to a new start to her career. She was finally able to wear the white dress, the white cap, a stethoscope round her neck and the nice smile that would keep germs and pain away from the children and people. She indeed enjoyed her work as a nurse and the smile never left.

"Do you imagine nurses abroad have better pay and better benefits than us?" One of her colleagues volunteered the information as they were having lunch. "… In fact, they are given better benefits than us including tuition fees to advance their education, and I hear all you need is to pass their nursing board exam. The moment you land you get a job immediately. Actually you can hold two to three jobs. More so they pay in dollars. Do you know how much a dollar is exchanging for right now?" Another colleague interjected. "No! imagine the Nurses do not need two jobs; with one job they are able to (doing a finger count) pay all their bills, pay school fees for relatives back home, build houses and get rich. I tell you America is the place to be!" She said with finality. A third one came up with the evidence. "I have a cousin of mine who went in for a one and a half year nursing program. As we speak he is (doing a finger count) earning so much money, he has built a house for his parents, is educating his siblings and he has been sponsored to advance to a degree level." There was silence in the lunch room as everyone internalized the discussion wondering if they needed to venture into the idea of going abroad or not.

Later that week at a family dinner, Nancy's uncle came up and told her. "You know if you went abroad you would earn more money with your degree than you are now?" Her uncle proceeded to tell her few of the success stories he had heard and witnessed. He added the fact that some people had resulted into changing their career to nursing. Nancy was astonished by this information. "How can two different people bring the same topic around the same time?" Nancy thought to herself. "Take your time, research and think about it. Then you decide your way forward." Her uncle told her.

Nancy did further research and convinced herself she would give it a try. Nancy got a sponsoring agency, who promised her they would process her documentation. All she needed was to send certified high school and University certificates and pay processing fee so that they can start the application process. Six months later she had sent the needed certificates, as well as paid the agency its dues. When she did not hear from them after six months, she started smelling a rat. Further investigations revealed that; the state she sent the certificate was legitimate, unfortunately, the stated agency was not. Their web page was now down. This frustrated Nancy very much, but she did not give up. She decided while she looked forward to getting a job, she might as well enroll for a Master's program.

With her education background, Nancy was able to get a scholarship to one of the Universities to pursue her Masters in Nursing and carrying her dream of making it into the American healthcare workforce, she said the sad good byes to her friends, neighbors and family and boarded the plane to the place with 'greener pastures.'

Upon arrival, she had to first settle down, then report to her new school and finally, start her journey to being a nurse. She searched for the website of the agency that had promised her a smooth transition. She confirmed, the website was non-existent and accepted that she had been conned. When she informed her host about the website, her host told her, "Those fake nursing agencies have really conned many people. When nurses are applying to agencies like this one, they need to check their credibility. Relatives and friends need to confirm the information they give instead of narrating the 'kitchen talk'. Now, forget the past and start over, this time contact the board of Nursing directly. I forbid you to use those agencies again!" Nancy took a walk as she contemplated the eye opener she just got. "At least there is still a chance to start over." she encouraged herself.

Meanwhile at home, everyone was waiting to hear the progress of the daughter of the soil. The church that had zealously prayed for Nancy awaited for her to give her dues, the people who had loaned her money to process this or that started getting impatient and the phone was ringing off the hook. She was a newcomer in one country, and felt like a financial refugee from hers. These were very disturbing times in her life. She could not gather the courage to talk to her father and explain the situation. She believed she was a big girl and she would handle the situation very well.

She started the process of sending both high school and University certificates and licenses verification from the country of her initial training. Her transcripts had to be verified and translated to the American system to ensure that the Nursing preparation she had gotten was up to par with the American standards of Nurse preparation. This process took a couple of months which were both frustrating and tiresome. It was at this point that Nancy realized that she was a foreign nurse and this was not her territory. She contemplated on returning home, but, she had already started her Master's program which had broadened her mind and she had gotten few ideas of her own on how she would contribute to the Nursing career.

"Good morning Nursing board how may I help you? Can I have your first name please? The representative politely replied. "My Name is Nancy Wa..." Excuse me ma'am, I did not get your first name. Could you spell it please?" Nancy was getting impatient now. However she started. "N... A... N... C...Y..." "Okay thank you. Let me see if I got all the letters correctly, then you can proceed to spelling your second name. Alright N...E...M..." Nancy had to interject. "No No No... It is N for No, A for Apple, N again for No, C for Cat Meow! Meow! And Y for You." The representative, with relief in her voice, replied "Oh Nancy. Okay let us proceed to second name." Nancy interjected "Before we proceed I would like..." This time was Nancy's turn to make nursing board representative repeat the sentence as she was talking too fast. While the representative was having trouble talking to Nancy, Nancy on the other side was frustrated because the representatives was talking too fast for her to understand. This was one long conversation but Nancy and the representative tried to be as professional as possible. The important thing at this juncture was to ensure both parties were duly satisfied.

Nancy believed she was fluent in English. She came from a country where English is a language that is spoken from Kindergarten and considered an official language throughout the country. She did not think she or anyone else would have a problem with English. She discovered, the difference in phonetic transcription and articulation of words often occur in situations where the participants in a conversation speak different tongues.

While Nancy was battling the different cultures and tongues in a foreign land, back home people were expecting her to send money since she is in a 'lucrative profession'. They did not understand why the son of so and so or the daughter of so and so seemed to have 'hit the jackpot' while she was still struggling. Nancy had had it!! She finally made the most depressing call to her father, and explained her situation as it was and all that had transpired and explained to him that she was not able to be like the sons and daughters of his friends who seemed to have 'hit the jackpot' when they landed to the United States. Nancy's father understood the situation and promised to work with her to get her settled as soon as possible. The process of sending and verifying transcripts and licenses took longer than expected. Her family was fed up with this new conquest of greener pastures and they wanted their daughter home at whatever cost. Nancy then decided to complete her Master's program and head home.

Finally, the certificates were verified, all of them with the right information and correctly signed, all she could do was sigh and await the verdict from the nursing board. "Good morning Nancy, this is your friend Salma I wanted to inform you that it is best you start preparing for the exam as you await the verdict of the Nursing board." Nancy was not sure whether the wintery weather and sub-zero temperatures were better than the news her friend had just given her. She replied in a somber tone "Okay. How, where and, when do we start reading for THIS exam?" Salma noticed her somber tone. "Okay! Girl! Okay! It is not as bad as you think. Just read any book that gives tips on how to pass the Nursing exam. Read cover to cover then go and seat for the exam. You will pass." Nancy went to the book store and purchased a nursing exam book and she started reading it and doing the test questions. "Hey, it's Jabulani, how is the exam reading coming along?" Nancy answered, "Not so bad, I have this book I bought, my friend told me it will help." "Oh no no no not that book? Mhhh it will not help, go take it back and take this other one." Jabulani interjected. "Ah!! Jabulani, am almost halfway done with this one, are you sure about that one you are telling me?" "Hee Nancie, all those years you have known me, have I ever lied to you? My cousin used it and he passed that exam. Go buy it or you will have to reseat that exam and it is stressful woo woo! Actually, I have it, I will send it to you. Give me your address. Make sure you read cover to cover." For the Nth time, Nancy wondered what she had signed up for.

Nancy finally got her authorization to test (ATT). This was another shock to her. "It is not guaranteed that you will seat for your exams despite having all your certificates and documentations correct. You have to be given the authorization to test (ATT)?" She registered for the test, continued reading hard, reduced number of visits, prayed hard, and built up her confidence. She had never failed an exam in nursing school. Nancy eventually sat for the test. She was confident about passing the test. She could not wait for the results. She had already bought the scrubs, a stethoscope and had started practicing her smile that had faded with everything going on.

As the bright sun rays looked forward to warming the wintery weather, she browsed the website to see if she had passed. She could not believe what she saw, her eyes opened wide her mouth wider yet no sound came out. You would think the snow had fallen on her face and melted away. All she could see on the screen was 'FAILED THE TEST' A cloud that did not have a silver lining overcame her. How would she explain to her host, her family, and her friends that she had not made it? Her debts were piling up, her savings were going down, her host was becoming impatient. Almost one year has been lost preparing for this exam, money, energy and all she would harvest was a 'FAILED THE TEST'? Nancy could not hold back tears of pain and frustrations. The tears could only be compared to the rains of the Congo forest; you could touch the darkness that befell her life. Nancy was convinced she needed to see a counselor. She took a month or so to recover from the shock. After which she resolved she will not quit with first failure. She will rise up, forge forward with renewed hope and conquer this exam.

She talked to one of her professors who informed her of various programs that give tutorial services to foreign educated nurses in order to pass the nursing exam. These programs are offered either online or on site. With a bruised ego, a drained account and renewed heart she purchased the tutorial program, and started preparing for the exam afresh. She had to keep away from her very 'reassuring friends' for a while and concentrate with the one advise she got from someone who is in the academia.

These sessions helped Nancy not only to study for the test, but also transition into the American Nursing system. She again dedicated her time to working towards passing the exam. She had to go through the process of being issued another Authorization to Test (ATT). She sat for the Nursing exam. The sun had finally shone. Her dawn had come. This time she was happy and she celebrated the victory with her family and friends.

The next step was to look for a job. Getting the license was the first step of the transition. She had passed many hurdles. This made her developed a 'Never say die' attitude. This would help her with the rest of the transition. Her smile that was once lighted, then dulled, was now out shining more than ever. She was ready to heal and heal she would.

The transition process should always start from when one makes the decision to move. So that one is able to provide the relevant documents individually as opposed to waiting for someone to do it for you. Always rise before a fall.

Chapter 2
URIAH: At the Acme

"I am very conscious of the fact that you can't do it alone. It's teamwork. When you do it alone you run the risk that when you are no longer there nobody else will do it"

Wangari Maathai

There comes a time in our lives we get fed up with the harsh situations we were born into. This gives us motivation to work hard to get out of them and be better people and hopefully pull a few others as we climb to the top. Climbing to the top is a journey that requires insight, determination and the right attitude to overcome the hurdles we find on our way. It also requires the right network and personal decision not to be swayed no matter how colorful the curb looks.

However, there is the struggle of getting ideas on what to do next after one reaches to the top of the ladder. This is a struggle that many nurses who leave the country and are able to make a better living or further their education in the foreign land encounter.

When not handled well, this part of success may turn into a bitter and regretful situation.

As nurses, we should look forward to nurturing and mentoring those who come behind us. Giving them correct information and guiding them towards the right direction as opposed to the usual saying that 'nurses eat their young'. In addition to nurturing and mentoring the young, we should also step in and mentor those who want to venture into other areas. As much as nursing is a noble career it cannot stand by itself. As thus, it is of paramount importance for nurses to thrive in multidisciplinary teamwork.

We should never forget where we came from. As much as we work hard to get out of these harsh environments we were raised in, we need to go back and help raise the standard of the place. That is give back to the community.

Uriah

Uriah was an ambitious young man and had an inner urge to change his life, and that of his family. His mother had worked hard to put him and his four siblings through school. During holidays, Uriah would do minimum wage jobs so as to help with some household bills. Although Uriah got some play time, it was not as much as his friends since he had other responsibilities. Being able to balance playtime, working minimum wage jobs during holidays and making good grades in school, resulted to Uriah growing up being a responsible boy as well as a mentor to his siblings. His mother made sure Uriah and his siblings followed the stipulated time table, did their homework and, prepared for the next day. They excelled in school and once in a while they would be awarded scholarships. This not only eased the burden of Uriah's mother on the tuition fee, but also created more time for Uriah and his siblings to study and enjoy their childhood. Due to school fees issues, Uriah was not able to attend a well-equipped high school and this posed a challenge to his future career. However, despite these difficulties, he did the best he could.

Unfortunately, he was not selected to join the University in any category due to his grades after high school. The urge to improve his life was still alive within him and was pushed by his great need to change his future and that of his family. In order to do so, Uriah needed to join a career that had a steady income, thrived in the competitive world, and would help him progress professionally. He therefore enrolled at the local Missionary Nursing School where he studied nursing. He graduated with a diploma or associates degree in Nursing. Being a local resident, he was absorbed into the payroll at the Missionary Hospital. Some of his friends who had migrated to the city encouraged him to relocate to the city in order to get a job with a good company or a bigger hospital. Uriah was tempted to go, but he was due for a promotion. Furthermore, his siblings needed him closer home to mentor them and his mother appreciated the help he offered. However he put it at the back of his mind he would relocate one day and experience working in other places.

While at the mission hospital, some missionaries came to visit both the school and hospital. As the head of his department, he was able to interact with the missionaries. During some discussion sessions, he discovered that he would actually be able to pursue a Bachelors of Science in Nursing. "I would be interested in pursuing a degree in nursing abroad. I would be glad to know how to go about it and the challenges I am likely to face." Uriah enquired from one of the nurses who had been sponsored to go abroad and had returned. The returned nurse candidly explained to him, "Your biggest challenge would be coming back home after spending years in training." Uriah did not understand the challenge and the responsibility that going in for a higher degree bore; especially to the people he would have to leave behind.

"You see, many people hope to come back and build the place they left but due to challenges, affiliations and/or influences they decide not to come back, or are forced to stay longer than they want or need to. There are others who make big promises that they do not intend to keep and are too ashamed to come back."

Mmmmh! Sighed Uriah. "So what would I need to do to avoid that trap?" The nurse explained to him, "First make sure you look for some form of funding, second make up your mind to come home after training, third do not make any promises to any one, forth make sure you go fulfill your purpose, fifth, expand your network with people from various backgrounds and cultures. Finally, learn as much as you can and think of ways you would implement those lessons here. You can make it if you try hard enough." Mmmmm! Uriah sighed again.

Uriah had just had a good bite of some food for thought. As the sun was setting, he went to his favorite spot besides the quite river to meditate. As the moon light and the stars escorted him home in the cool night, Uriah's brain was boiling with thoughts. At dawn as the sunshine spread its rays in the sky that morning and burst into the horizon, Uriah spread his blue print across the table and saw endless possibilities. He would do it.

The next day Uriah sat down with one of the missionary nurses who explained to him the process of getting a scholarship and the many challenges involved in studying abroad. Uriah followed the stipulations and was able to get to everything he needed. He was guided on how to apply, where to send his transcripts and certificates. After the good byes and promises of a better life, Uriah boarded the plane to America.

Upon arrival, it did not take him long to get approved and issued with the Authorization to Test. Unfortunately he was not ready to test. His advisor advised him to take the online tutoring program so that he would be able to transition to American Nursing as well as get practice on the exam. At the completion of the tutorial session that took him a couple of months, his feet were swollen and his bottom was sore but he had passed his nursing exam. His friends and family were very happy and celebrated with him.

The next thing was for him to look for a job. He already had put in some hours working as a nurse. He had even worked as unit manager at the missionary hospital so for him, he believed it would be easy to get a nursing job. He worked on his resume to make it as presentable as possible. To his dismay, when he went to take his resume he discovered that there are pre-made application and all one needed was to fill the necessary information. He went around filling applications in any and every healthcare facility.

Then he waited to be called. 'Hey Uriah, how are you doing? Did you apply at my work place? They are hiring." His friend informed him. "Yes I did but they have not called me yet." Uriah replied. "Okay, if they do not call you at the end of the week, call them and tell them you applied" His friend advised and hanged up. Uriah waited for the week to end and a second one went by. Uriah started calling the various places he had applied to. Some of them said they were not hiring at the given time. One of the calls revealed that he did not have the American experience as a nurse and that had hindered him from getting hired. He resolved to network with some foreign trained nurses to help him navigate the job market.

Soon after he got a job as a nurse, he noticed that his friends had increased in number as well as calls from home asking for money. At first this was not hard to handle. However, he realized that he had an academic responsibility to keep his grades up or he would lose his scholarship. Unfortunately, this revelation came after he got an academic probation for one of his classes that he realized his entire life was at stake. He had to do something drastic or he would have to forfeit his scholarship and wave his dreams good bye. With renewed insight, Uriah reduced the number of friends and had to change his circle of friends to people who would mentor him to be a better person. In addition, he had to regulate and minimize hours at his work place. This worked well for him since he was able to attain and maintain good grades in school till he graduated with his Bachelors of Science in Nursing degree.

When he was done with his Bachelors of Science in Nursing there was celebration both at home and his current stay. Once he graduated with his Bachelor of Science in Nursing degree, he had a battle within himself on whether to go home or live in America. He compared the healthcare system and financial remunerations. After a long discussion with one of his mentors, Uriah decided to stay back and help people back home upon request. He proceeded to do his Masters in Nursing and was able to sponsor his siblings and some relatives to attend school till University level as well as mentor several young people in his village. He actively participated in raising funds for both the Hospital and the School back in his hometown so that it can better serve the community.

After completing his Masters of Science degree, he went back to his blue print. This time he had the clarity he needed. It was time for him to go back home and do all he was doing but at close proximity. He went back home and started community based health projects, helped in areas of sanitation, clean water for every household, wrote some proposals which helped equip both the hospital and the nursing school with state of the art equipment and simulation machines. He lectures some classes in the school, but mainly deals with administration and mentoring of the young people.

Uriah started life at what most people would consider disadvantaged level. He however did not give up his dream despite the hurdles he had to face growing up. When he got to the top, he did not forget the village that raised him up and he gave back to society. His aim was to better his life and that of his family but he ended up making life better for his whole village.

Chapter 3

RICHARD: Making Informed Decisions

> *"He who knows nothing is closer to the truth than the one who is filled with falsehoods and errors."*
>
> *Thomas Jefferson*

To many people, first world countries seem to be the beacon of hope for their existence. When one gets a chance to board the flight that will take them to any of the first world countries, they go at it blindly without researching about their host countries. Upon arrival, they discover the difference between a mirage and an oasis.

Getting the right information before venturing out is of paramount importance. It helps to simulate what happens in reality and the knowledge on how to handle the situation effectively. One's source of information is also important: One needs to get information from people who have been in the same situation either directly or indirectly. This would entail having mentors or peers who are knowledgeable about life in the diaspora.

It is of paramount importance to verify the information given by either going to the website or by communicating via e-mail or phone call to the respective places and affiliates. When one gets to know the truth, it is philanthropic to share these truths with others.

Richard

Richard came from a family of people who were well educated and had travelled in and out of the country for education, business and leisure. Consequently, upon completion of his high school education, Richard knew his destiny was to live, work and learn abroad. He had dreamt about it many times and had confided this to some of his friends who also had similar dreams. However, his bubble was shattered when his parents told him he had to get a degree from Kenya first before proceeding to any other country.

Richard believed that his parents were being plain stubborn and did not want him to enjoy his young life. However, his parents knew the numerous challenges that students face abroad. His father had spent three years abroad one of which he was a student and worked for two; His mother had joined him during his last one and a half year. They had worked in various countries before settling down in their native country. This experience put Richard's parents in a good position to advise their son to get some basic skills in his home country before going out into the world. Inside him he did not approve of it, he was actually angry at his parents and at the world in general. He had seen a number of his high school classmates board the plane to a new land. A first (fast) world country!

His parents did the philanthropic thing and held a seminar that targeted parents who were taking their children abroad at such a young age as well as parents whose children were abroad. They made a power point presentation on the life abroad. They highlighted the challenges these children face despite being hosted by their family or friends abroad, the delicate balance between work, play, responsibilities, school, socio-cultural challenges and how they affect their lifestyle, their personal development, social lives, as well as other things like climate change, culture shock among other things. He also emphasized the importance of parental guidance during the first years of their college life on choice of friends, finances, and lifestyle. After this presentation, to the dismay of their children, some parents made the decision to take their children to local colleges while others decided to take the risk and send their children abroad.

After completing his studies, he did his one year Nurse internship, and prepared to meet his friends, pass the dreaded nursing exam, transition to American nursing, work in America, and eventually join a master's program. Richard had a plan. Therefore after passing the Nursing exam, he joined the hundreds of other foreign trained nurses in the journey of looking for a job in America. Unfortunately for him, all the facilities he went to needed someone with not only nursing experience but also nursing experience in American health care. Despite the fact that Richard had worked with patients of various ages and illnesses, adding to the fact that research had shown there was a great healthcare out cry due to shortage of nurses; information which had been confirmed by his friends and relatives who worked in the industry. He could not get a job right away.

He continued applying and hoping there will be an opening and worked in any job that would accept him. It took him four to five months to land a job, which hired him as a new graduate since he did not have any American nursing experience. Having no other option, Richard took the job.

As he trained in the job he discovered that nursing knowledge and skills were similar. However, culture, equipment, types of disease and illness were new to him. While in training, he encountered more of tropical diseases and less lifestyle diseases. His new job offered him more lifestyle related diseases and less tropical diseases. He also realized he needed orientation to use the ever improving equipment and evolving technology the facility was bringing in. He also needed to adapt to a certain company culture while working with people. He also noticed there were more men pursuing nursing. Richard was ready to learn all the new things that came his way. This opened doors to places that he had never thought possible. Richard was able to attain certification in various nursing skills like Cardiac pulmonary Resuscitation (CPR) instructor, parenteral therapy amongst others. He eventually decided to advance his practice in Cardiology a specialty he enjoyed studying and working in.

Choosing his specialty came almost natural to him. He was able to get to the right school, the scholarship he needed and of course the right attitude. This, he did swiftly with minimal conflict with his parents as well as with himself. Richard had the right information, the right guidance to ensure he reached his goal swiftly.

As an immigrant nurse, one has the advantage of having a taste of both worlds. The knowledge and skills learnt do not change, they only improve with time. The challenges are best overcome when the person has a positive attitude, is ready to learn as well as mentor the ones coming behind them. The nursing knowledge and skills taught do not change; however, the situation and disease processes have variations. Therefore, the immigrant nurse should be confident of the knowledge and skills they have acquired and be ready to learn ways in which they can be implemented in the new environment.

CHAPTER 4

SALLY: Accreditation of Schools

*"Be sure you put your feet in the right place,
then stand firm."*

Abraham Lincoln

It is a common believe that one can enroll into any institution of higher learning as long as it offers what an individual desires to pursue and have a friendly fee structure. However, there are schools that have not met the requirements of the board of education in the listed country thus they are not accredited. This comes with greater disadvantage for students in a non-accredited institution of higher learning compared to those who attend an accredited institution of higher learning.

When it comes to choosing schools or institutions of higher learning, ensure you get people who have gone through the same process directly or indirectly. It is good to have a large network of people who can give you different experiences.

The advantage of having academic qualifications from an accredited institution is that an employer can trust the quality of skills and knowledge being employed in their business. Even when one decides to venture into business ownership, they are confident of the knowledge and skills they are employing and have a reliable network of fellow alumni. In addition, these schools are streamlined in a way to ensure that the education is dispensed by quality and experienced lecturers. When the Alumni of these institutions get the top positions, they tend to hire a fellow Alumni or an Alumni of a institution similar to theirs.

Sally

Growing up, Sally was a very ambitious girl and wanted to follow in the footsteps of her auntie who was also her role model. Auntie Sharon was a professor at the local public University and had recently, attained her Doctorate degree in Chemistry. Sally's mother was working on enrolling for a Doctoral program. Sally's dad had attained a Master's in Business and held several certificates. Not only did Sally and her siblings have people to mentor them but also gave them a reason to follow these three great examples of academic achievers. Sally, being the first born, wanted to create a path for her siblings to follow. She was passionate about education and was ready to get to the top.

After completing her Bachelors of Science in Nursing, she worked in different nursing departments in various capacities. When Sally was working as a nurse manager she made a decision to advance her career. She started searching for Universities she could enroll to. She narrowed her search to Universities that offered scholarships, friendly eligibility criteria, and a maximum of two entry exams. As she was buried in the search engines, her friend came and informed her there was a school that did not have many entry level requirements and had affordable school fees. Sally jumped on the chance to enroll into the school, she downloaded all the information needed and excitedly went to inform her Auntie Sharon she had found a school that would help her realize her dreams.

Auntie Sharon read through all the papers and requirements. The facial expressions could tell the story of her findings. Her facial expressions changed from, "I am proud of you daughter, smile" to "I cannot believe this!! …" Sally who had been watching her all this time was baffled at the behavior exhibited by her Aunt. With questioning eyes she looked at her Aunt for answers. Without a word, Auntie Sharon walked to the computer, and ran some data base that Sally could not understand. Her Aunt moved from one data base to another, this left Sally with more questions than answers. She tried to follow what her aunt was doing to no avail. Sally decided to go get herself a cup of water when her aunt started talking. "The school you are applying to is not accredited." Auntie Sharon broke the silence in the room. "Okay, and what does that have to do with me and going to school? That should be the school's right problem." Sally thought to herself, but politely asked her aunt. "What does that mean and how will it affect me and my school?" Her niece was not alone in this category. Many students, both local and international, do not know the difference let alone the importance of attending an accredited school for advanced level of studies.

Auntie Sharon sat her niece down and explained importance of attending an accredited institution of higher learning. "Accreditation of school means that the institution has met the stipulated requirements set by the country's education board. This ensures these institutions give quality education to its students and confers valid degrees. As thus, if you graduate from a non-accredited institution of higher learning, your degree is not valid and your chances of getting a job will be diminished, if not nullified." All Sally could do was sigh with disbelief.

Sally enquired with a surprised face, "How do you know a school is accredited?" Aunt Sharon opened the computer to the database she was searching. Then she told her niece; "There are different ways of knowing. First, there are different accreditation agencies some will have a list of accredited institutions in the country, or a certain region in the world. So make sure when searching for institution of higher learning you look at all of them. You can never be too sure of it. Second, the institution should declare that they are accredited. You can call to ask or check from their website. Third, though not very reliable, you can ask the alumni of the institution, alternatively you can research where they are employed." At the end of the explanation, Sally was glad that she had someone who would guide her. Her Auntie looked at her and told her 'take heart my child; this is but a lesson to learn. Now what you do is search for an accredited institution of higher learning, tell your friend to do the same."

Sally went ahead and started looking for an accredited school with a good reputation to pursue her Master's degree. Her friend did the same too and this gave them a better and satisfying experience both as students and employees. She has since encountered people who went to non-accredited institutions of higher learning and seen the frustrations they have had to endure as they tried to validate their degrees. Some had to go back to an accredited institution of higher learning in order to be able to work on their dreams.

Looking for a school to pursue your career at an institution of higher learning is a process that requires personal research, advice from people who have gone through the system, and verification of the credibility of the school. The degree you pursue is usually as credible as the institution you attend. In addition, one should always verify the information given using all the possible resources available. Had Sarah not verified the information from her friend with her aunt, she would have ended up joining a non-accredited school, which she would have regretted.

Chapter 5

ERIC: Gender Based Careers – stereotype or reality

Nurses serve their patients in the most important capacities. We know that they serve as our first lines of communication when something goes wrong or when we are concerned about health.

Lois Capps

There comes a time in one's life when you are the only one who can comprehend your dreams. The passion and excitement of this dream may not be understood by people until they see it in fruition. This is because everyone has a bias toward certain things in life depending on the environment, culture and life experiences. One's dream surpasses all these dependent variables and incapacitates the mindsets of people who believe these dependent variables are viable.

From time in memorial, gender based roles have been clearly defined and strictly upheld. This has trickled into career choices.

Some careers are male dominated, and others female dominated. This paves way for the largely acquired and accepted belief that there are careers exclusively for men while others are exclusively for women. When one decides to go into a career dominated by the opposite sex, they face discrimination from even members of their own gender. However, if you hold onto your dreams and passion for your career choice, the environment will soon harmonize with you and more people will eventually accept you and your career choice.

'Men in Nursing' is a topic that has been debated since the first day a man joined Nursing school. Many men face discrimination from their fellow men due to the fact that it is largely accepted as a career exclusively for women. Some of the female nurses, members of the interdisciplinary team and patients discriminate the male nurses. However, it should be noted that Nursing has many specialties and both men and women have a choice of going into any of them. Nursing is a unique career that has continued to develop in terms of technology, autonomy and quality. It has created its own path that the fore-founders would be proud of. It is paramount to note there is an increase in number of genuine male nurses. It is therefore important to support the male child in his career choice as a nurse.

Eric's Story:

Eric's greatest dream was to change his life and that of his family since childhood. He constantly prayed to God to help him achieve it. He was a very bright young man who unfortunately lacked the resources for a good education. However, he kept his dream alive and focused on being nothing but the best. School fee was a great struggle for him let alone the extra tuition fee, for after school tuition. To survive, Eric had to sell some few items like mangoes and oranges after school till dusk when he returned home to do his studies and assignments before the tilly lamp wick burned up or the oil dried up. As he walked around the village selling his products, he noticed there were many buildings in the area but one essential one lacked - a healthcare facility. This created an inner urge in him to be a nurse and put up a healthcare facility so that he can help children and adults get medical help. He knew right away he wanted to be a community health nurse. Eric knew it would take him more effort than his peers, but he resolved he would make it. He had to make it.

When Eric did his final year of primary school; he was among the top fifty students nationwide. He was admitted to one of the most prestigious boy's high school. He knew he would not make it because his mother would not afford to gather enough money for his high school and he did not have enough time to work for the amount of money needed. Fortunately, since a child belongs to the village, the villagers pooled their resources and networks together and Eric was able to attend high school all the way to his fourth year and was able to graduate top of his class. This enabled him into be admitted to the Nursing department of one of the nation's top Universities. He was excited!! He had not only taken a second trophy home, but also had come closer to realizing his dreams. For this, He thanked God in the way he knew best.

Eric was elated when he went home to share this great news of his admission to the Nursing program at one of the top universities in the country. "I made it to the University! I made it to the University!" He jumped with excitement as he entered into the family compound. "Aririri! Aririri!" his mother ululated as she went to meet him halfway into the compound. Other family members and neighbors streamed into the compound with every woman joining in the ululations. "Aririri Aririri! Aririri! Our son has done us well! Aririri!"

The ululations blared as the visitors to their compound brought the ABCs of victory: Admiration, Blessing and Congratulatory messages. School children were rushed and others dragged into the compound to see this second time hero. Eric was the hero they needed to emulate. The old people came to spit their blessings. Then the familiar village chorister burst into song and dance which everyone joined in and the compound suddenly turned into a dance arena. Its was such a joyous moment for everyone. When the songs calmed down, the crowd started walking away to their various duties with both jeers and cheers showing in their face.

The family was finally alone. Still in high spirits, Eric's mother enquired about the program. "I am in for nursing! I will be a nurse!! Yeeeeee!"......He jumped up again, as he was in midair, he looked at the faces of his siblings and mother. You would have thought a catastrophe had just happened. His mother's face was like a flame of wildfire engulfing a forest. Eric's younger sister asked him, "How can you study Nursing? Nursing is not for boys it for girls!" he immediately knew why his mother's face was a fiery furnace. There was grave silence the remainder of the evening. Cold ash had just been poured on their spirits.

The next morning, Eric's mother shared the news of her son to Eric's uncle and soon news was spreading through the village like a wildfire. Some of Eric's friends bantered him for being in a career believed to be for women. With the new revelation, Eric's heroism started fading away. He was caught between his dream career and that of his family. He reasoned he would get solace from the other young men he had graduated high school with and had chosen nursing as a career.

When he met his friends from school, half of them had changed their majors from Nursing to other Majors like dentistry and medicine. Ninety percent of them for the same reason "Nursing is a career for women." Others asked him, "How can you bend down to clean and bandage wounds?" He was surprised at the fact that many people regarded nursing as a career pursued or meant to be pursued by only women. Well his dream mattered and he decided he would go to the ends of the world to ensure that he had achieved his dream. He reminded himself that everyone may not get it now, but later when health care has been brought close to them, they will appreciate it. By now he knew many people will not appreciate him as a person. He needed to be strong for himself.

Upon completion, Eric was employed as a staff nurse in one of the hospitals. That was where real lessons on how the workplace and society viewed the male nurse started. His nurse manager, a female nurse, would always allocate heavy or hard-to-deal with patients to Eric and other male nurses. If a patient suffered a bout of psychosis, or were too violent, or too heavy, Eric and other male nurses were expected to naturally take care of these patients. Eric noticed the younger patients and nurses were not alarmed that he had decided to be a nurse. However, most of the older patients believed he was a doctor and often confused him with the doctors. Some of his male patients enquired of him why he had chosen to be in a female dominated profession and laughed it off telling him he will have a mindset of a woman. Most of the female patients, especially the older women, were not comfortable being treated by a male nurse especially when it came to things like assessment and baths. The more time Eric spent with the patients, the more they became receptive of him. "Our son Eric cannot be in a career meant for women. This is an abomination." You would hear neighbors whispering. "These young men of today do not know how to be men." The lamentations were endless.

After gaining some nursing experience, Eric decided to work on his dream to be a community health nurse. His dream was alive and burning right inside of him and was few steps away from achieving it. Envisioning his dream coming true right in front of his eyes caused goose bumps – that is what is called passion. However, there was a cloud that hanged over his mind about the reaction of the villagers to the Health Center he had planned to build. Would they reject the Health Center the way they had rejected his decision to be a nurse? Eric still had the challenge of being in the minority count at his work place. How was he going to convince not only his mother and the whole village but also his new friends and fellow female nurses that men can also make good nurses?

After working for one and a half years he won the green card lottery and was able to relocate to America. Life would have never worked better. He would be able to work, save and come back home and build his dream hospital in his village. Before he left, his uncle called him for a man-to-man talk. They discussed culture, his role and responsibilities in the family, amongst others. The biggest of them being the fact that he will need to change his career to a more male oriented one. "Eric, you are a bright young man and you can start a new career. So when you get to that land far away, change that career of yours and study one that befits a man of your stature!" His uncle told him as he playfully thumped

Eric's chest and then nods. "Blessings as you explore the new lands son."

On his plane ride across the oceans and continents, Eric wondered what the new land had for a male nurse. His dream of being a community nurse still hung on and there was no way he was letting it go! He had worked too hard, endured too much and his passion for the career had grown too high. Eric landed in America, passed his Nursing Board exam, got a license and after a while, got a job as an Emergency Room Nurse. He was on high alert on how the rest of the staff and the community in this new world viewed male nurses and how they would treat him.

He discovered that nursing was still viewed as a 'female career.' However, due to mixed cultures and economic situations, the number of male nurses was higher than in his homeland and male nurses were moderately accepted. He noticed a majority of male nurses had actually changed from the 'male careers' into nursing. Half of them held down the job because of economic reasons while the other half accepted and loved their career move.

Eric decided to make a comparison on the two worlds - Kenya and America. Both worlds viewed nursing as a 'career for women', men are gradually getting into the career mostly due to economic reasons, and job security, the younger patients were more accepting of male nurses more than the older generation, nursing staff managers in both worlds are happy to have the male nurse so that they can help with stronger patients and do the 'hard' stuff in the unit. Eric noticed male nurses from societies that have a rich culture and strict traditions were fewer. This made Eric conclude that culture and traditions have a very strong influence over men choosing nursing as a career. This has made many men to get into careers where they are suffering economically and lack passion in so long as they are 'male oriented' careers.

When he was done with his Masters of Science in Community Education and Health promotion, Eric went back to his village and started a Health Center that offered essential health services and health education. He was accepted by his family as well as the villagers. He still wonders about the real reason they accepted him back. Was it because they finally accepted that a man can be a nurse or was it because of the services he was providing? Those were answers he did not want to investigate. He was living his dream and he would be building himself.

Eric used the networks he formed both abroad and at home to upgrade the health center which is slowly evolving into a regional hospital. His resilience in a career that is branded as a 'women only' career has changed his life, his family's, and more importantly, that of his community. He has also empowered several other people to go into the career of their choice as opposed to what is deemed 'fit' for them to pursue. This has seen some ladies from Eric's village go into careers that are male dominated and men into careers that are female dominated and fit in well. His persistence and following his dream has broken the strong believe that 'Nursing is only for women.'

Times have changed and we need to embrace the positive changes. We should not let obstacles or certain mindsets prevent us from attaining our goals and dreams. In addition to that, on average people spend at least eight (8) hours of their day working. It is therefore important to choose a career where one enjoys spending eight hours of their daily life.

Conclusion

Many people will have a dream and may not achieve it because of various challenges they face along the way. However, there is always a path that is open for the people who are determined to get to where they want to go, and have a passion for what they want to do.

When one finds their niche' in nursing and decides to start their journey as a nurse, they will need to realize it is not a linear journey. There are many obstacles and challenges that will come along this journey. Some will be exciting, some will be dulling, and some surprising; the good news is that these are part of the learning process. These progressive nurses will also need to know it is not one of those careers you retire from. Once a person is inducted as a nurse, you will always be.

Nurses have always immigrated from country to country, continent to continent due to various reasons. However, the recent years has seen many nurses migrate from third world countries to first world countries. The move to migrate is usually challenging to the immigrant nurse, however, the remuneration and recognition they get in the foreign country is above what they get in their home country. This leaves their home country with less educated, less trained and less mentored nurses. Consequently, there is a great outcry from these countries and the healthcare system for the nurses to relocate back and fill the big gaps they left.

This may be difficult to achieve due to logistics and dynamics that are beyond the control of the immigrant nurse. However, the immigrant nurses should pool resources, network and help the healthcare system that trained them to reach their goal as nurses.

As one decides to relocate, it is of paramount importance to have a strategy and true, verifiable information about the process of relocation to ensure a smooth transition. After making the decision to migrate, one should first contact the board of nursing of ones intended place of relocation and ask for the academic and professional requirements and, where to send them. there are documents that will need to be verified by the CGFNS Commission on Graduates of Foreign Nursing Schools, while others are sent to the State board of nursing, type of test accepted in the State and waiting time for evaluation of documents. This will help the intending immigrant nurse to send these requirements themselves as opposed to waiting for someone else to do it on their behalf, reduce frustration and anxiety. In the meantime, the intending immigrant nurse should look for a reliable Nursing exam tutorial program, as they wait for the verification and approval of their documents. This can be done as the immigrant nurse is preparing to relocate.

Respect is a two way street. As much as we expect our culture to be respected, we should respect other people's culture. Culture shock is one of the things that we face once we move from our cultural comforts. Immigrant nurses will experience different work place cultures and work ethics. These should be respected and adapted slowly. Diversity is accepted but one should learn the system first and see where one can enrich the system and enhance teamwork.

Most immigrant nurses are known to be hard working and dedicated to their job. The zeal they put into building their careers and adhering to work ethics is to be applauded. However, this should also be used to mentor and encourage the upcoming nurses back in their country of origin. As well as help in development and support therein nursing societies created.

www.ingramcontent.com/pod-product-compliance
Lightning Source LLC
Chambersburg PA
CBHW021047180526
45163CB00005B/2314